Calm Mind

–

Healthy Body

Discover How to Calm Your Mind,
Improve Your Health
and
Take Back Control of Your Life

RON KNESS

Contents

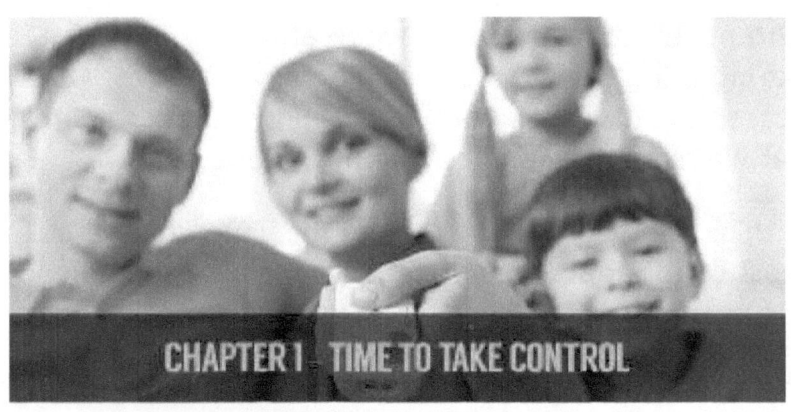

CHAPTER 1 - TIME TO TAKE CONTROL

Chapter 1: Time to Take Control

Do you ever get the feeling like you're constantly putting out fires? Like life is one massive struggle to stay afloat?

Do you come home from work feeling tired and stressed and without the energy to do anything other than collapse in front of the TV?

Do you always feel like you're just *not quite* as happy as you think you could/should be?

That's life my friend in today's world. Or at least it's life as many of us have come to know it. In fact though, there's no reason this should necessarily be the case.

The problem is we're always chasing after the gold at the end of the rainbow and in doing so, we end up chasing out tail and take the time to stop and smell the roses.

Sorry to mix metaphors, but I feel it paints a fairly accurate picture of the situation today for most of us.

We're never happy because we're always striving for "the next big thing" and what is coming next. We're always stressed about what's coming up and we never appreciate what we have here and now until we lose it.

We think the only way to change this is to change our lives. To work harder and longer, which in the end only adds to the problem.

But it's not. The way we change this is from the *inside* out. We need to change the way we think about our situation and we need to change the way we approach life's problems and the way we enjoy the moment.

And that means taking control of our individual minds. Once you can do that, you can take back control and you can feel confident, relaxed and happy in the exact same circumstances. Once you can do that, you can start creating the space to actually plot a course and to start changing life for the better. You can stop treading water and actually start swimming.

All very abstract, yes. So far it sounds like a platitude from a bumper sticker.

But stick with me, because this is where the science comes in. And it might just change the way you think about your life, your brain and the interplay between the two.

It's Your Perception That Matters

Think about it this way: it's not the situation that matters, it's your perception of the situation that matters.

And I mean this in the most literal and realistic of senses.

Think about it this way: you can be surrounded by fire and be completely calm and happy, or you can be relaxing at home and be completely stressed.

In the first case scenario, you're surrounded by fire but you believe you're invincible. As far as you're concerned, nothing can hurt you and you have nothing to fear. As a result, you remain calm and your heart rate doesn't even rise (well, other than from the effects of the heat!).

In the second scenario, you're sitting at home, comfortable and with a warm cup of tea. You're surrounded by family who love you and you have the TV on showing your favorite TV program. But all you can think about is the work you have to do tomorrow, your money problems and the fact that you're not as well off and as successful as you'd like to be.

As a result, your body and brain interpret the signals as you being in danger. Your brain produces more norepinephrine, more cortisol, more dopamine and more adrenaline. As a result, the person who is surrounded by flames but deluded is actually happier and calmer than the person who is sat at home but stressing out.

Now of course I'm *not* saying that you should be like the deluded guy surrounded by fire... That's dangerous!

But you also really shouldn't be like the stressed guy who should be relaxed. And here's the thing: lots of us are!

THIS is why it's so important to start taking control of your mind. Because it's what will impact on your happiness, your calm, your focus and on all the other things that contribute to you being happy and successful.

Changing your environment and circumstances is often incredibly difficult – nigh impossible even – but you can change your *mind* today. And that can bring incredible benefits.

Identifying the Issue - Stress

A stressor can be anything that increases your "fight or flight" response. This response occurs when external or internal stressors cause the body's adrenal glands to put out excess epinephrine, norepinephrine, and cortisol. These response hormones can result in an increased heart rate, respiratory rate, blood pressure, and blood glucose levels.

A stressor can be anything from having a bad day at the office, relationship issues, physical or emotional distress, financial problems, and a whole host of other things that infiltrate our daily lives, resulting in a stress response. Stress is normal but too much of it, or too often, can lead to negative effects on your health.

Stress is actually a normal part of life. Without stress, we cannot respond to the demands of our daily lives. And unknown to many, stress can be brought on by good life experiences as well as bad. Stress is both a physiological response and an emotional response. The physiological response is that which was described above. The adrenal glands put out hormones that cause physiological changes in the body.

The emotional response to stress can be excessive anxiety, anger, dissociation, or frustration. While you may have more energy under stress, stress has a way of causing mental and emotional changes in the brain that can interfere with concentration, memory, and overall emotional well-being.

Stress can be caused by something physical, such as being exposed to an overwhelming danger, or emotional, like worrying about finances, work or relationships.

Common causes of stress include the following:

- Internal stressors

- Survival Stressors

- Overwork and fatigue

- Environmental Stressors

Effects Of Stress On The Body

Stress has a way of causing bodily changes that can eventually result in premature aging and fatigue. Some common ways stress affects the body include the following:

- Decrease in cognitive ability

- Appetite Changes

- Insomnia

- Decreased sex drive

- Physical pain

- Dental Pain

- Loss of hair

- Unusual behaviors

- Nightmares and strange dreams

- Twitching of the eyelids

Physical Conditions Related to Stress

Stress can cause physical conditions that can negatively affect the quality of your life. Here are a few common diseases that can be traced back to excessive stress affect your physical body:

Weight gain. Stress can cause you to crave foods higher in calories, sugar, and fat. When under stress, you are more likely to choose junk and highly processed foods that are easy to just pick up and eat. There is more to the picture, however. In a research study out of the journal

Biological Psychiatry, women who faced at least one stressful event during the previous day burned more than a hundred fewer calories after eating a fast-food dinner as opposed to women who at the same dinner but were not under stress. This may not sound like much but it translates into an extra eleven pounds in any given year. Years of stress can lead to obesity, related both to food choices and to changes in metabolism. Stress hormones can increase insulin levels and will decrease the oxidation of fat, which promotes the storage of fat. Increases in bodily cortisol levels are also linked to an increase in fat around the belly. As you get older, the metabolism begins to slow naturally, often resulting in weight gain.

When you add to this problem by allowing stress to cause overweight or obesity, you become even more vulnerable to a host of chronic disease in old age, including, heart disease, type 2 diabetes and stroke.

Colds and flus. Research has been done on people under stress and the incidence of them getting colds and flus. In one 2012 study, researchers asked 276 healthy individuals about the types of stress in their life and then allowed them to be exposed to a type of cold virus. Those who were under chronic stress were resistant to cortisol and were more likely to catch the cold when exposed to the virus. The same phenomenon is believed to affect a person's ability to catch the flu. Cortisol affects the immune system, putting you at a greater risk of catching bacterial and viral illnesses.

Poor wound healing. When under stress, cortisol in the body causes poor wound healing. It can also decrease the effectiveness of vaccinations, particularly in the elderly population or in people who care for them. There is research indicating that women who must care for their elderly relative suffering from dementia take nearly 10 days longer to heal from a wound when compared to those women who weren't caregivers and under that type of stress. The longer the stress continues, the more disrupted the wound healing response. Having strong social bonds that decrease stress can improve wound healing.

Sleep disorders. There is less restful sleep in people who are under stress. Stress can cause you to awaken more often during the night and can cause early morning wakening. This is especially true in the aging population.

Because a lack of sleep results in poor emotional control and memory loss, those who cannot sleep may find it more difficult to deal with life's stressors, further increasing the stress a person experiences. Increased cortisol levels can result in waking up more at night, resulting in rumination about stress instead of sleeping.

Cardiovascular disease. There is an increased risk of having a heart attack and being under stress. One research study, published in *Nature Medicine*, discovered that blood taken from stressed-out medical residents had high levels of white blood cells that can lead to inflammation and heart disease. Cortisol causes white blood cells to alter their texture so that they attach themselves to a greater degree to the walls of blood vessels. This increases plaque formation so that heart attacks are more likely. This has also been proven to occur in non-human studies. Since heart disease is the #1 killer of both men and women, especially in their senior years, it is more important than ever to not allow stress to contribute to this epidemic.

Stomach Problems. For the last half century, doctors believed that stomach ulcers were related only to stress. Then it was discovered that a microorganism (Helicobacter pylori) contributed to stomach ulcers. On the other hand, about 15 percent of stomach ulcers happen in individuals who do not have the microorganism in their system. Only about 10 percent of those infected with H. pylori actually get ulcers. It is theorized that chronic stress affects the immune system's ability to handle H. pylori, resulting in ulcers. This puts stress back in the running as a cause of stomach problems. Stress can also lead to heartburn, ulcerative colitis, Crohn's disease, indigestion, and irritable bowel syndrome.

Pain in the Neck, Back and Shoulders. Too many people spend much of their days huddled in front of a computer, laptop, or iPhone. This can lead to an increase in back pain, neck pain, and shoulder pain. It also leads to physical inactivity and strain on the brain that can worsen the pain. Pain in the musculoskeletal system is generally more related to stress in the workplace than to anything else. Inflammation secondary to stress can interfere with healing of the minor tears and spasm involved in back, neck, and shoulder pain.

Mental Conditions Related To Stress

Stress can contribute to a variety of mental conditions as well. Some of these include the following:

Depression. Stress can lead to changes in the neurochemicals of the brain so that depression is more likely to occur. Decreases in serotonin, norepinephrine, and dopamine can adversely affect sleep, libido, appetite, and mood. It has been found that individuals who are severely affected by depression have chronically elevated levels of cortisol, which can negatively affect the function of the hippocampus and can cause permanent damage to the brain cells.

Cognitive changes. Stress can bring about changes in memory and other cognitive skills. Those under chronic stress have a decreased ability to remember things and often suffer from poor concentration.

Anxiety. Stress can bring about an increase in anxiety. The body responds to epinephrine and norepinephrine by increasing the neurochemicals in the brain associated with anxious symptoms.

All in all, it is easy to see how too much stress can adversely affect your health. In the rest of this book we are going to explore ways to calm your mind thus reducing stress down to manageable levels, improving your physical and mental health along the way. Let's start our journey to mental and physical wellness!

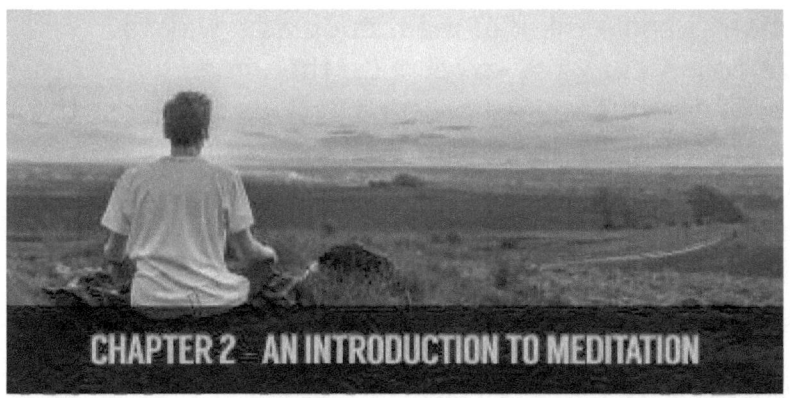

Chapter 2: An Introduction to Meditation

When we think of taking control of our minds and finding calm in a busy and hectic world, many of us will instantly think of meditation.

Meditation is an ancient practice used by billions of people around the world and one that has been practiced for centuries. Now scientists and researchers are starting to decode it's many benefits but nevertheless, it's still very understood by a great number of people.

Let's take a closer look at meditation, how it can help us and how you should get started.

Just What is Meditation?

Perhaps a good place to start is to answer the question: what *is* meditation?

While many people think of meditation as a way to 'achieve enlightenment', to recreate the effects of hallucinogenic drugs, or to practice various religions; the reality is that meditation is simply a form of practicing control over your thoughts. It *can* be all those other things, but at its most basic root, meditation means try to focus your thoughts or clear your mind, which is essentially the equivalent of training your attention.

So often our thoughts are reactive instead of proactive. We are constantly being distracted and taken from one experience to the next – whether due to television, to music or to something else entirely. But when you meditate, you will be actively *controlling* your thoughts. You will become introspective and you will start to reflect on the very nature of thought itself. And as you do, you'll learn to remain in control of your thought processes so as to prevent yourself from becoming easily distracted, stressed, angry or otherwise experiencing inappropriate or unhelpful emotions.

This is a *highly* valuable form of training and one that's particularly relevant in today's fast-paced and constantly-connected world. Meditation can help us conquer stress and improve concentration in a range of tasks.

The Varied Benefits of Meditation

Studies show that meditation can help us improve our mood, our concentration, our focus, our creativity and more. It has both *immediate* benefits by providing us with a break from the stress of our internal monolog and helping us to experience 'theta brainwaves' but it also has long term benefits as we start to learn to better control and understand our own thoughts and emotions.

Meditation has *even* been shown to boost our IQ! That's right, it can actually make you *smarter.* And this also correlates with more connective tissue in the brain and a greater ability to utilize different areas of the brain at once for single tasks.

Fortunately, meditation is gradually starting to make its way into the mainstream. More and more 'productivity' and 'lifestyle' coaches are recommending its benefits and it forms an integral part of Cognitive Behavioral Therapy (CBT) – which is currently the most popular form of clinical intervention for a whole host of psychological difficulties.

Still not convinced? Then I invite you to have a listen to Tim Ferriss' podcasts. Tim Ferriss is the author of *The Four Hour Workweek* and is one of the most influential writers on the net when it comes to topics like fitness, self-improvement, productivity and happiness. His most recent project – the podcast – sees him interviewing a large number of different influential figures. Those include Matt Mullenweg (creator of WordPress), Maria Popova (of Brain Pickings), Arnold Schwarzenegger and many, *many* more. One of the questions he'll often ask them is what their morning routine looks like and if they have any other habits they consider important to their success.

What does Tim Ferriss note is the *one* thing that nearly *all* his interviewees have in common? They all meditate. So if you want to be one of the world's most influential entrepreneurs, if you want to be spiritually enlightened or if you just want to be *smarter,* then you need to start meditating!

But while meditation has benefits across the board, it's worth noting that *some* forms of meditation appear to be more effective at promoting specific physiological benefits than others (according to a study from the National University of Singapore). If you want to get the best benefits from meditation, then you need to choose the right type to get started with.

Here's what the study found when comparing Theravada and Vajrayana meditation...

Theravada Meditation

In the study from the National University of Singapore, it was found that Theravada meditation is more effective than Vajrayana (below) for promoting relaxation and calmness. Studies measured activity of the parasympathetic nervous system – the prime purpose of which is to promote calmness – while practitioners were deep in meditation.

Vajrayana Meditation

Those using Vajrayana meanwhile were found to activate their sympathetic nervous systems, which control the fight-or-flight response. In short, this would lead to elevated heartrate, focus and arousal. This is a particularly interesting finding, as conventionally we view meditation as a means to calm ourselves and to relax.

After the participants had engaged in their meditative practices, both groups were then asked to take cognitive tests and it was found that the Theravada group were able to boost their performance considerably from a single session. The same boost in cognitive performance was *not* seen in those using Vajrayana meditation.

This demonstrates the broadness of the term 'meditation' and shows that different types of meditation have different specific advantages. In this scenario, you might decide to use Vajrayana meditation to psych yourself up for a competition or to prepare for an interview, then use Theravada meditation to calm down afterwards or to chill out before bed.

The Different Types of Meditation

As you can see then, the type of meditation you use is a very important factor in determining the outcome. Likewise, you will likely find that some forms of meditation are more accessible and enjoyable than others, depending on your own goals, your experience and your interests.

The question then becomes: where to start? Read on and we'll look at some different types of meditation and some different terms. Bear in mind that you don't have to stick rigidly to any one of these and actually you can create your own 'kind' of meditation by just setting your own goals. Nevertheless, any of these will provide you with a good starting point to do more of your own research and to start practicing the art of meditation.

Mindfulness: Mindfulness, also called 'Vipassana', is a type of meditation that comes from Buddhism. It's also the form of meditation that's perhaps most widely used in the Western world today – a good example being its use within CBT (this is something we're going to come to in much more detail in subsequent chapters).

Essentially, the goal in Mindfulness is to be 'aware' and to be 'present' of your own thoughts and to reflect on them.

This form of meditation doesn't encourage you to try and empty your mind then, but rather the objective is simply to let your thoughts 'drift by' like clouds in the sky.

What this then allows you to do, is to become more aware of what thoughts you actually tend to have, thereby being better able to spot negative thought patterns that might be causing problems. This type of meditation has also been shown to reduce anxiety, almost as effectively as anxiety-reducing drugs. Perhaps the biggest advantage of mindfulness though, is that it's not as challenging as trying to completely empty your mind of thoughts and thus provides a great starting point for those interested in learning.

Zazen: Zazen is a term that essentially means 'seated meditation' and is sometimes referred to by the modern Zen tradition as 'just sitting'. This is an incredibly minimalist sort of meditation, which once again makes it ideal for those interested in getting started by feeling a little anxious to give it a go. The *only* instruction here is to sit with the correct posture, meaning that there's no pressure to get anything 'right'. The simple act of sitting completely still is almost sure to result in a calming effect and to gradually clear your mind, thus there is no need for complex instruction beyond 'just sitting'.

While this is the core principle behind Zazen, it will sometimes be more complex than that. Often practitioners are given a paradoxical sentence, a story, a question or an element of Buddhist scripture to 'muse on'. This method of meditation has also been adopted by a number of other religions – whereby believers are asked to think about lines from their respective religious scripts, or to think over scenes from their literature.

For some, the lack of guidance is going to make this an approachable and enjoyable form of meditation, for others it can be frustrating and might leave you lost.

Spiritual Meditation: Another way in which meditation has been adopted by religions is through spiritual meditation. This is essentially a form of meditative prayer – and prayer has been shown to have many similar benefits to other forms of meditation.

Transcendental Meditation: Transcendental meditation comes from Vedanta, which is the meditative tradition from Hinduism. TM starts out seated (ideally in lotus or half-lotus position) and this time uses a mantra. A mantra is any word or sound of your choice, which is simply repeated over and over again. The idea behind this form of meditation is simply to 'rise above' any distractions or thoughts, effectively clearing your mind of all thoughts and living entirely in the moment. Alternatively, you can try focusing on your breathing in order to calm your thoughts.

The ultimate objective of transcendental meditation is transcendence. This is the meditation that is used as a path to 'enlightenment' which is reportedly a feeling of 'oneness' with the universe and perfect contentment. In reality, it's likely that enlightenment is merely a brain state, achieved by relaxing areas of the brain and thus getting them to shut down. This is something that takes years to master though and is highly elusive, if you use transcendental meditation with the sole objective of reaching this kind of state, you a likely to be disappointed.

That said though, if you can reach this state, the effect is something similar to being on drugs or having a stroke.

It's completely mind-bending but not damaging in the same way those other examples are. You lose the ability to distinguish time and to distinguish your own body in physical space as those areas of your brain close down. If you want to have an 'end goal', then this is certainly something interesting to aim for.

When done correctly, transcendental meditation is ideal as a way to relax and to move your thoughts away from stress. It can be used to calm the heart rate and is a fantastic 'coping mechanism' if you suffer with anxiety. It's also quite difficult though and many people give up after becoming frustrated at the inability to quiet their inner voice. The secret to success is to go easy on yourself and not to force it.

Focused Meditation: As with transcendental/mantra meditation, focused meditation involves the practice of trying to completely clear your thoughts by focusing on something else. Mantra meditation is one form of focused meditation, but you could alternatively try focusing on external stimuli (like the sound of a river, or a piece of meditative music), or even on something like a candle flame.

Guided Visualization: Guided visualization is a form of meditation wherein the practitioner visualizes a scenario or environment. The 'guided' part of this process involves listening to a recording, which often will describe the scene you are in. This kind of meditation is great for relaxing and for moving your thoughts away from the hustle and bustle of daily life, before you achieve the ability to block out your surroundings through other forms of meditation.

If you're feeling stressed and you want to immediately calm down, then guided visualization is a useful tool. However, it doesn't require the same discipline as other forms of meditation and so is not likely to help develop your ability to focus or to calm yourself in the same way.

Movement Meditation: In movement meditation, you relax your mind while focusing on your body and moving through a range of gentle movements. A great example of this is Tai Chi Chuan, which is a martial art practiced incredibly slowly involving a set of gentle movements. While it takes time to learn something like a Tai Chi set, you can practice movement meditation by using a dance routine (Solja Boy?) or even by just swaying gently from side-to-side.

Vipassana: Vipassana is 'insight meditation' (Vipassana is Theravada meditation, Theravada being a branch of Buddhism). This is meditation which involves 'close attention to sensation' with the goal being to discover 'the nature of existence'. This form of meditation comes from Buddhism and was believed to be the type practiced by 'Buddha himself'.

To practice this form of meditation, you sit down and then focus on your abdomen and feel the way that the breathing moves your stomach. Likewise, be aware of the other sensations throughout your body, trying to remain focused and calm simultaneously. When interruptions come – such as sounds, other thoughts, or temperatures, you should 'note' those sensations and give them labels such as 'warmth' or 'thinking'. Vipassana is often practiced on retreats, where participants alternate between seated and walking meditation.

Vajrayana: Vajrayana is another branch of Buddhism. Vajrayana meditation is a complicated and advanced form of meditation, which involves the goal of becoming 'buddha' like. There are various types of meditation within Vajrayana, such as Mahamudra. This form of meditation involves attempts to empty the mind once again, this time by simply 'doing nothing' to the extent where you aren't even focused on trying to meditate.

Both the Theravada and Vajrayana forms of meditation are advanced methods and require years of practice to perfect and an understanding of the surrounding beliefs and cultures. They are also only two examples of the many complex and varied forms of meditation that exist.

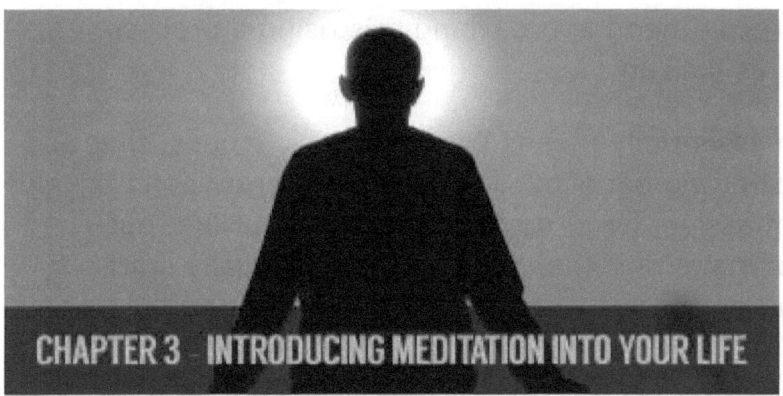

CHAPTER 3 - INTRODUCING MEDITATION INTO YOUR LIFE

Chapter 3: Introducing Meditation Into Your Life

So that's the general concept of meditation. The next question is: how do you start adopting it into your routine and making it a part of your life?

Because this is the part a lot of people will struggle with. In fact, there's a better than average chance that you've already tried to get into the habit of meditating, only to find yourself giving up quickly because 'nothing is happening'.

This time, we're going to get it right.

A Simple Program to Get Started With

For most people, starting with mindfulness, Zazen or transcendental/mantra meditation is advised. These are perhaps the simplest methods you can use when you're just learning and will help you to get a great start to your day every morning.

I also recommend approaching this using a process known as 'kaizen'.

Kaizen essentially means 'lots of small changes, that add up to offer big benefits'. The idea is that you don't try and make massive, large-scale changes in your life, but instead make tiny changes and then gradually start building on those.

For instance, trying to go to the gym five times a week, for an hour at a time, is often an up-hill struggle and is something a lot of people will struggle to stick with.

Going for an extra 5 minute walk or doing some sit-ups every other day though? These are things you can much more likely do and continue doing. And once you start doing that, it will be much easier to throw in some press ups, or to extend that walk to 10 minutes.

So this is the best way to start gradually introducing meditation into your regime: with very small and easy chunks of time.

Start with Zazen – sitting meditation. Take *5 minutes* every morning to just sit and relax with your eyes closed. No goal, no stress and no trouble. You might find you can even do this while your partner is in the shower, or by waking up five minutes earlier. Almost all of us can find some time in the day for five minutes of quiet.

Aim to do this for 2 weeks with no other goal than to sit quietly every morning for that amount of time. Don't expect anything to happen and don't expect to 'feel' anything.

From there, you may want to progress to actually having a goal. You can aim to make this goal a better awareness of yourself (by using mindfulness) or you can aim to quiet your mind and learn to block out stressful thoughts (by using transcendental meditation).

I recommend aiming for both. Perhaps try increasing your time to 10 minutes and spending 5 minutes on mindfulness and 5 minutes on transcendental.

I personally find looking at a candle flame to be *incredibly* helpful when practicing transcendental meditation. However, it is entirely up to you how you do it.

Just know that even when you're aiming to quiet your mind, you should never be 'punitive' and you should never punish yourself for not managing to achieve your goals. If you find that your thoughts are wondering or you're being distracted, just *notice* that it has happened and let yourself be calm and focused again.

The reason it is *so* important not to have a strict aim or to reprimand yourself for getting it wrong, is that this introduces stress to what should be an innately calming activity.

At this point though, you're now starting to enjoy meditation as part of your everyday life and that means you should have formed the positive habit (remember, it takes 30 days to form or break a habit). Now you can see what works for you and start learning more/experimenting.

Using Tools and Getting Help

Still struggling to get into the swing of things? Another option is to try guided meditation. Guided meditation means that you'll be following a set of instructions that will be spoken verbally. You can get these as a sound file or as a video and the idea is that you listen to them and follow the instructions in order to clear your mind/observe your thoughts.

Because this gives you something external to guide you, it makes it much easier not to let your mind wander. A great place to look for guided meditation is on YouTube – but you can also try the excellent 'Headspace' app.

Another option is to get help from someone who knows what they're doing. An easy way to do this is to go to a class such as yoga or Tai Chi, where you will likely have some guided meditation at the end of sessions.

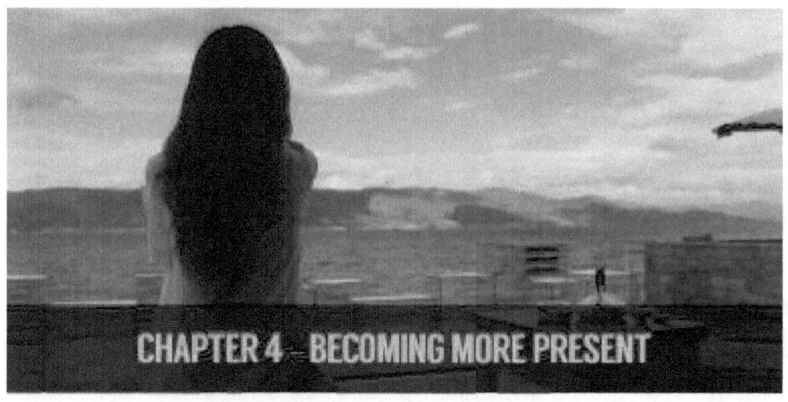

CHAPTER 4 – BECOMING MORE PRESENT

Chapter 4: Becoming More Present - Meditation in Everything You Do

There is no 'end goal' in meditation but one vague aim is to get good enough at meditating that you can eventually clear your mind or *detach* from your thoughts at will.

This way, you can then prevent yourself from being distracted by unwanted thoughts whenever you want.

I like to call this 'bubble time'. Bubble Time is the name for the small 'segments' of time I give myself throughout the day when I can be completely relaxed. I'm in a mental bubble and able to block out all activity outside my bubble.

Imagine that you have a very stressful day and you've been working hard through a massive to-do list. You need to make lots of calls, manage your work team and just generally deal with a lot of fires.

Plus you have a date tonight with someone that you think will be awkward and you have pressing, on-going money concerns. Sound familiar?

Anyway, you're going home on the train and in that time *there is no benefit to being stressed*. In other words, you can carry on worrying about all those things you have to do tomorrow if you want to... but it's not going to do you any good. What would be *far* preferable, would be if you use this short amount of time as a break in order to recuperate.

Now if you've never practiced meditation, you're going to struggle to do that.

But if you haven't? Then you can put yourself in a meditative state and become indifferent to that stress. You can sit back and just clear your mind. Now, when you arrive home, you're going to be much more recharged and energized because your brain has had the opportunity to get some rest. The result is that you'll feel much better and you'll enjoy your time at the end of the day much better as well.

If you get *really* good at this, then you can eventually start to employ 'moving meditation' as in Tai Chi. Except now, you're going to be in a meditative and relaxed, focused state at the same time as walking, talking and doing other things. You'll be impervious to stress because you've learned to *control* your mind and *control* your emotions.

Because you aren't giving your concerns the emotional weight that you may have done in the past, your brain isn't activating the 'salience network' that it uses to respond to threats and you're able to just carry on going about your business in a completely calm and efficient manner!

Being More Present

Meditation is one way to stop worrying about all those little nagging concerns and doubts. Another way though is just to become more present and more in the moment.

How can you do this? One method is to start focusing on your body and on your senses a little more.

The fact of the matter is that most of us are so *in our own heads* that we barely notice half of what's going on around us. We walk in a dream state worrying about work, or about our relationships and we hardly take the time to stop and smell the roses – literally *or* metaphorically.

Try this right now. Turn off any music that you're listening too and instead just start to notice the sounds around you. Really listen! What can you hear? Perhaps the hum of traffic outside? Maybe the murmur of conversation in the room? Maybe you can hear next door?

Or perhaps you're outside? Maybe you can hear the sound of birds?

Likewise, you can probably smell a whole load of things you hadn't noticed. And if you take the moment to feel your own body, then you can probably notice the sensation of the seat pushing into your legs and into your buttocks. Maybe you can feel the blood filling your face and making you feel hot. Or perhaps there's a cool wind blowing against you. What direction is it heading?

Likewise, listen to the sounds of your own breathing and feel your abdomen expand and shrink as you do.

Once you do this, you'll find that you stop worrying what's going on around you and that you start to appreciate your environment a little more. There's so much that you normally miss!

You can try doing this on walks too. Go for a walk with no music, no phone and nothing else and try just being present and noticing the world around you. It's a calming and invigorating experience at the same time!

Being More Present in Conversation

Practicing this is important because as with practicing meditation, it will eventually become something that you can just engage at will. Now you can choose when you want to start listening better to what people are saying to you and when you want to really focus on the day out you're having with your children.

Again, you can leave your work concerns at work.

And try focusing on the sensations of your body more the next time you're being intimate with a sexual partner.

Don't worry about your technique, what you're going to do next, whether they like you... instead, really *focus* on how the touch of their hand feels on your body. You'll find that you instinctively know what to do next and that you start to be much more passionate and responsive. You'll become a better lover, simply by getting out of your own head. And you'll feel it far more forcefully.

This is true for everything else as well. Next time you have a bath, take a moment to *really appreciate* the warmth and the softness of the water against your skin. Indulge yourself in the smell!

The next time you eat cereal in the morning, remind yourself how much you enjoy that cereal and how happy you are to *not* be going to work.

This is what so many of us don't do. So many of us are constantly in a dream state and worrying about other things that we actually miss what's going on around us.

Being stressed and having no control over your mind is doubly problematic – because not only does it make us unhappy directly but it also distracts us from the things going on around us *all the time* that could be making us happier.

Oh and what this does for our relationships is also *fantastic*. Right now, being distracted by work could well be destroying your relationship with your family and friends.

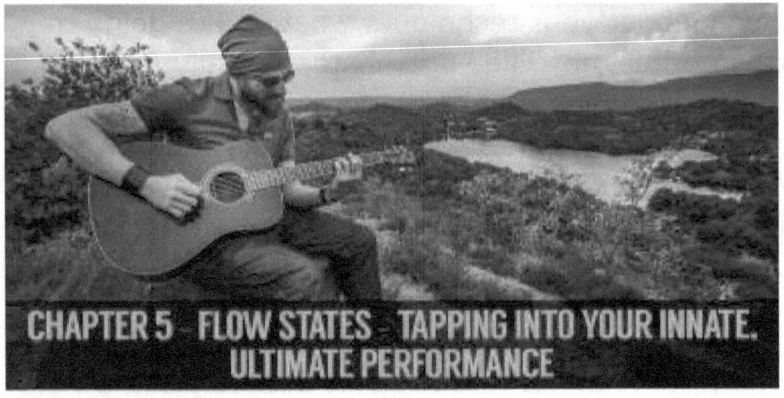

Chapter 5: Flow States – Tapping into Your Innate, Ultimate Performance

In the first half of this book, we've learned how to use meditation and how to start introducing it gently into our lives. Now you have the ability to focus at will, to stop feeling stressed and to actually control how you feel and what you want to think about. This is an incredibly power because it means that you can choose to actually live in the moment and you can choose what's important to you and how you want to feel.

But what if I told you that this isn't just about 'happiness'? What if I told you that this is also about getting the very most out of yourself. What if I told you that the things you've just learned could help you to tap into your full potential and to become almost superhuman?

Do I have your attention?

Welcome to 'flow states'.

How to Stop Being a Zombie

Remember what I just said about the importance of focusing on what's going on around you? And on being awake, alive and in the moment?

This is how we're *supposed* to function all the time. This is how animals and babies are all the time. Somewhere along the lines, we lose that connection with our environment.

The question you might now be wanting to ask is: why is it so hard then, to do the thing that we were designed to do? Why is it so hard to obtain the same focus and connection with the world that comes naturally to infants?

There are lots of answers to that question but one of the most pertinent is that we are too set into our routines and we aren't stimulated enough or stimulated by the wrong things.

Try that exercise again where you listen to your surroundings. What can you hear? Can you hear a ticking clock somewhere?

There's a good chance that the answer is yes if you're indoors but you might not have noticed it until I asked you to listen to it. And why not? Because you've become desensitized to it.

What's happened is that your brain has heard that ticking before. It's the exact same every second and it's something you're completely used to.

As such, your brain says 'this isn't important' and it pushes it into the background.

Meanwhile, the worries that are flooding through your mind constantly seem *very* important.

The same thing happens if you cut ping pong balls in half and place them on your eyes. When you do this, you'll at first see the insides of those ping pong balls, as you would expect. But after a few minutes, things will go fuzzy.

Why? Because nothing is changing. The nerve endings in your eyes have become tired of the exact same stimulation and so they're turning off. Nothing is moving, nothing is changing – it's inefficient for them to keep firing.

This is called the 'Ganzfield' experiment and it's quite interesting if you ever want to induce hallucinations naturally.

Now think about what you do in your daily life:

- You walk the same route to work

- You take the same ride on the same bus

- You have the same breakfast

- You have the same conversation with the same people

- You perform the same tasks throughout work

- You get home and sit in the same place

Guys... this is killing us. Our brain has a complete lack of stimulation and excitement from this kind of activity. We evolved to be constantly moving, constantly in danger, tracking our prey through the wild... and when that happened *everything* around us seemed important, dangerous and salient.

But now, we're sleepwalking through life. Everything is safe and everything is the same...

If you want to be more present and more in-the-moment, then you need to submit yourself to environments and situations that are exciting, novel, different and interesting.

If you do this, then you'll *automatically* forget all those things that are making you stressed. You'll *automatically* become more engaged with the world and less worried about your own petty concerns.

So take different routes home from work.

Learn new skills and hobbies.

Have conversations with strangers.

Try new foods.

When you do, your brain will light up and come alive and you'll get a reprieve from your money and relationship problems. Better yet, you'll form new neural connections which will once again help you to become sharper, smarter, faster, more creative and more **alive**.

What is a Flow State?

If the idea of subjecting yourself to novel states – or 'rich environments' – sounds familiar, then you may have read *Rise of Superman: Decoding the Science of Ultimate Human Performance* by Steven Kotler.

In that book, Steven describes what is known as a 'flow state' in detail. This is the condition in which we are most alive, most happy and the best at performing.

It's the exact *opposite* of wandering around and being stressed about work.

In a flow state, you are *so* engaged with the surroundings and what's happening that you forget 'yourself' entirely. Sound familiar? It's almost like a form of meditation, except this time you are completely switched onto the world around you.

This is something that most of us have experienced at some time in our lives and you may be familiar with it even if you think back.

Have you ever dropped something out of a cupboard and moved so fast to catch it that you didn't even think?

Have you ever been playing sports, when suddenly the world seemed to slow down to a crawl and you were able to move with superhuman reflexes and break your personal record with some kind of superhuman feet?

Have you ever been writing and been so engaged with what you're saying that you're able to completely lose track of time?

Have you ever been in a conversation that lasted all night?

All these are examples of flow states. And in fact, even watching a film can sometimes mimic flow. In this scenario, you might become so engrossed in what's happening on the screen, that you are shocked when you step outside and it's dark. It's almost like waking from a dream.

This is like 'action meditation' and it's thought to be at the heart of most of our scientific breakthroughs, most record breaking athletic accomplishments and all kinds of other examples of people acting their very best.

Flow States and the Human Brain

So what's going on inside that head of yours when you enter a flow state?

Essentially, a flow state is very similar to the 'fight or flight' response but with less 'negativity' you could say. It means that you think what is happening around you is very important and deserves *all* of your attention. As a result, your body starts to produce dopamine, norepinephrine, epinephrine, anandamide and other neurotransmitters. This causes your brain to become intensely focused, which creates the illusion that time has slowed down. You gain a kind of tunnel vision and now the only thing you're focused on is that one moment and the things you have to do to emerge from it victorious.

You begin to react almost automatically and instinctively with barely any input from your conscious mind.

And what this actually looks like in a brain scanner is called 'temporo-hypofrontality'. To translate that into English, this means that for a brief period of time, the front portion of your brain (prefrontal cortex) has shut down. This sounds like a bad thing until you realize that this is actually the part of your brain that's responsible for doubt and that slows you down.

When you're catching a ball, your body can do it perfectly every time. The problem is that you 'get in your own way'.

By letting the front part of your mind shut down in that moment, you can tap into the incredible reflexes and focus of your body and act on pure instinct. You become an incredible machine, capable of inhuman performance.

You break records in sports, you produce incredible work and you come out of it feeling alive and invigorated.

In fact, it is said that many people actually 'chase' after these kinds of flow states – and that this explains a lot of thrill seeking behavior.

Oh yeah and guess what temporo-hypofrontality also looks a lot like in a brain scan? You guessed it: meditation!

I *highly* recommend that you take up some kind of exciting hobby and that you start exploring more. Excite yourself and get yourself to focus and to pay attention!

The 'Default Mode Network'

Flow states are currently all the rage and are getting a huge amount of attention in the psychological literature as well as online, in forums and in popular culture. Flow states are being touted as the solution for 'everything' and as something we should strive to always encourage.

But actually, this is somewhat missing the point.

Yes, sometimes we should be alert and connected. Sometimes we should be able to shut out the outside noise and to focus on calmness, stillness and oneness.

But actually, that chatter and stress is not something we want to *entirely* eradicate.

Sounds like I'm contradicting myself now right? Stay with me!

Yes, when we were animalistic in our behavior, we were much happier, much less stressed and much more engaged with the world around us. But you know what? We were also *animals*.

We managed to achieve all those things that we achieved today by getting *out* of that reactive and engaged state and yes... stressing.

And not *all* stress is bad. 'Eustress' describes the kind of stress that motivates us to do things – things like perform our best at work, revise for exams, save money. Studies show that people who never feel stressed actually tend to perform worse in education and in their careers.

There's more too. Did you know that being completely focused is actually counterproductive to true creativity?

True creativity comes from letting the brain explore different neural connections – it is the act of recombining different ideas and memories into new formats and we tend to do this when daydreaming and when having an internal monologue.

When you do this, you enter what is called the 'default mode network'. This is exactly the state of mind that you're in when you are daydreaming and letting your thoughts run away with you. It tends to occur when you're engaged in mindless tasks – like commuting – and it too is responsible for some incredible breakthroughs. It's part of legend now that Einstein came up with the theory of special relativity while working in a patent office – and it was the dull and mundane nature of working in that environment that allowed him to do so.

It might be nice to think that flow states and meditation are the answer to everything – but they're not. They're actually just a very important part of our mental experience that many of us have forgotten. Instead of trying to completely eliminate one type of brain state, true control of the mind means being able to switch from *one* brain state to another with ease.

In other words, it means being able to mull over tasks and agenda items when you're a bit stressed or when you're working. It means entering a productive flow state when you're entering data, or when you're doing martial arts or sports after work. And it means being able to switch off and let your brain have some much-needed peace and quiet when you get home from work.

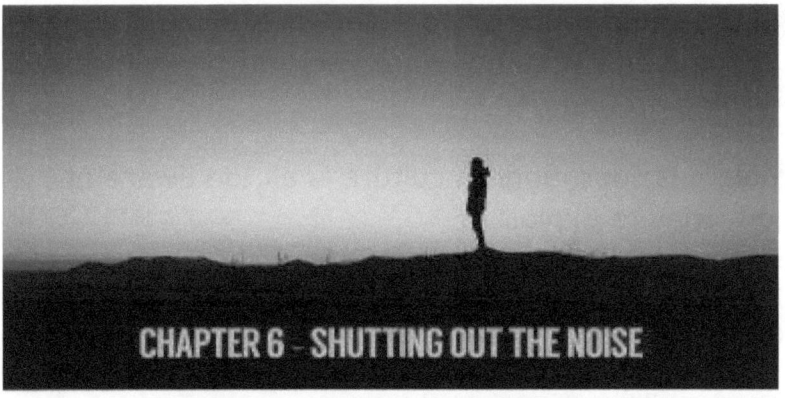

Chapter 6: Shutting Out the Noise

So the best type of mental state is the one that lets you switch to *other* mental states at will. Our aim is to be in control of our brains and our thoughts and to be able to switch from one state of mind to another with ease.

In other words? All types of thought and all types of mental state are important, valid and helpful.

Except one.

What is that one? It's the one where you're just incredibly distracted by all the constant demands being placed on you.

And *this* is where the 'modern ache' starts to come in.

Why We're Wired and Tired

Earlier, we learned how we were desensitized to much of the natural stimuli coming into our minds through our senses.

We take the same route to work and do the same things every day and as a result, we are very much desensitized to everything around us.

The problem is: our modern culture is all too aware of this and it tries to exploit it.

While you're happily mulling over the day's events you see, you're also being distracted by:

- Bright billboards and adverts

- Your phone's constant buzzing

- The TV

- The radio

- Your boss emailing your

- Cars honking their horns

- Alarms

- Computer games

All these things are designed to grab our attention and to over stimulate us so that they can get us to spend money/work/pay attention.

And this is what's killing our ability to focus, relax and concentrate as much as anything else.

Do you know why alarms are designed the way they are? They make a beeping noise because it's something we would never hear in the wild.

As such, it's strange and unusual to our brain and it sits up and takes notice – in comes that salience network and in comes that cortisol, norepinephrine and general *stress*.

And this is what wakes most of us up in the morning! We're startled awake from complete, deep sleep by a loud 'alien' sound.

Then what do we do? Normally, we will check our phones.

Bright light = even more cortisol (the stress hormone) being produced in our brains.

Then looking at adverts starts to grab our attention because that's what they're designed for.

Then we read our email. What's this? A message from your boss asking if you can do something for them as soon as you get in?

Now you're stressed and focused on that. And thus, as you do your teeth, it's all you can think about.

Over breakfast with the family, your mind is half-watching the television and this is preventing you from properly paying attention to what they're saying. The TV is much louder, much more colorful and is designed to grab attention.

What do we do on the way into work? Probably play a computer game. And those are all *about* making us pay attention. They stimulate stress by creating difficulty and when we do well, they reward us with the right sounds and colors. This creates a dopamine hit in our brain which is very rewarding and which makes the activity very addicting.

All this time we're missing the view out the window.

Then at work, we feel stressed again because we remember that email while we make coffee.

Coffee which – by the way – also triggers the release of more stress hormones.

Then we sit down and instead of doing the things we need to do first, we start our day by doing that thing that we were asked to do. Now we're in a 'reactive' state of mind and we're not able to do what's most productive or most important *for us*.

And so it continues for the rest of the day. We're constantly being tugged in every direction by computers, work, money problems, adverts, games, texts... and that's using up all our ability to pay attention, to focus and to think.

So is it any wonder that you're struggling to start meditating? Or that you're so 'wired and tired' all the time? Or that you're struggling to stay on top of things?

Using meditation will really help with this because it will give you the ability to control your focus and your ability to concentrate. Now you can say 'no' to worrying about that email. And you can say 'no' to focusing on the TV ads. And you can engage with your body and mind whenever you want in order to recharge and in order to start enjoying the world around you.

A Morning Ritual

What's also really good though, is if you can try and reduce all that noise, distraction, stimulation and chatter. This will just make everything easier for you and will help you to better focus on the things that matter to you.

One example of how you can do this is with your 'morning ritual'.

A morning ritual is basically a series of steps that you will endeavor to go through every single morning before you leave the house/start with work. This lets you stop being reactive and start being proactive. It means that you're now setting the pace and deciding how you want to begin your day – and it can help to make you more productive and efficient for the entire day that follows.

So what might a morning ritual look like?

Some great things to add:

- Read the morning paper – catch up on the news in a way that doesn't require the TV!

- 10 minutes of mediation

- No phone/email/computer until you get to work

- Do some exercise – 10-20 minutes is better than nothing and a great way to give yourself a surge of energy

- Healthy breakfast

- Write a to-do list – now you're taking control of how you're going to spend your morning/day instead

- Take a cold shower – it doesn't have to be cold but if you have the willpower to try it, you'll find it invigorates you, wakes you up and really helps you to focus and feel your own body

Similarly, you can also try introducing an evening routine. There are a few things this can help with:

- Write a journal – writing a journal is a great way to reflect on the day and how it could have been better/what you enjoyed about it

- No TV or phone for 30 minutes before bed – this will help to get your brain ready for sleep and will increase your production of the sleep hormone melatonin

- Read in bed – again, this helps you to feel sleepier and is also very meditative

- Have a warm bath – this can help relax the muscles for better sleep

- Lay out your clothes and/or gym kit for tomorrow

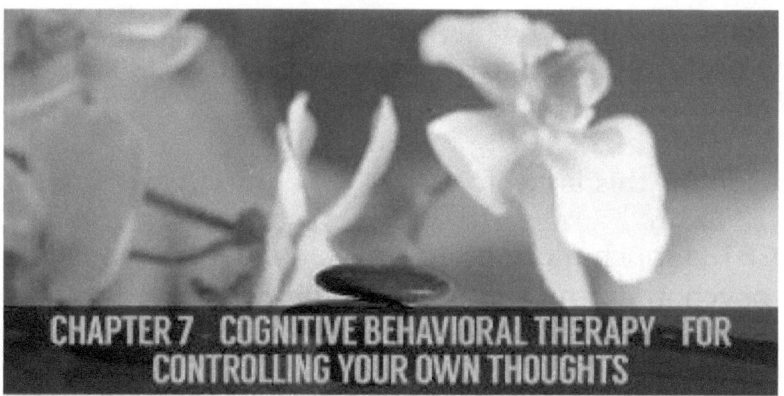

Chapter 7: Cognitive Behavioral Therapy – For Controlling Your Own Thoughts

Now you should be starting to get a better understanding of how your brain works, how all those distractions are negatively affecting it and how you can use meditation and 'flow' in order to start taking back control.

But you can go further with this and start engaging in whatever brain state you want at any given time. In order to do this, we're going to be looking at something called 'CBT' or 'Cognitive Behavioral Therapy'.

So exactly what is this?

What is CBT?

CBT is a psychotherapeutic technique. That is to say that it is a technique used by psychologists when they're trying to treat patients with anxiety disorders or with mental illnesses.

It is a framework that has become very popular and is now the preferred method of treatment on the UK's NHS and in many other health institutions.

The reason for this is twofold:

1. CBT is much more effective than older methods like 'psychotherapy' and has been demonstrated to work in a number of studies

2. CBT is quick, non-invasive and cost effective. It can even be used 'remotely' simply by sending the patient home to try and attempt on their own.

To understand what CBT is, it can be helpful to understand what cognitive psychology and behavioral psychology are individually.

Behavioral psychology is an old school of psychology that was big in the 50s. The central tenet here was that all our behavior and thought processes were learned through repetition, association and observation.

The most famous example of behaviorism in action is the study 'Pavlov's dogs'. Here, Pavlov demonstrated that he could get a dog to salivate when it heard a bell, simply by ringing the bell every time it got fed. Eventually, this 'classical conditioning' taught the dog to associate the bell strongly with the experience of getting fed.

Behaviorism attempted to explain every single aspect of our psychology this way. For instance, we learn to walk by learning to associate certain sensations with falling and others with success. And we learn our personality through reward and punishment from others.

Phobias and other psychological problems were the result of unhelpful associations forming and these could be treating by creating *new* associations.

Over time though, behaviorism began to lose favor as it appeared to over-simplify matters. In a strict behaviorist view of psychology, there is no room for our thought processes or our internal experience. What happens when someone plans out an action? What happens when we imagine something happening?

What about intention?

Cognitive psychology added this element in and looked at the brain more like a computer with a 'program' running. The program is our thought process and we use this to decide what to do and how we're going to do it.

CBT meanwhile elegantly combines both these approaches into one unified theory. We still learn through association but this can just as easily occur in our own heads. In other words, if you're convinced that you're going to fall off of a height, then you'll keep rehearsing it happening in your mind and you'll keep thinking to yourself that you're going to fall. This *alone* is enough to create the association and to make us afraid of heights.

So to treat a phobia, CBT will focus on reconditioning and creating new associations but it does this both physically and through changes to your internal monologue.

CBT Techniques Explained

So how might this work in practice? Generally, it involves several steps and several different techniques that when combined, allow you to control the way you think and feel.

The start is to identify the way you feel and what you're thinking when you're doing something...

Mindfulness

And guess what... this is where mindfulness comes back in!

Say you're afraid of public speaking and you want to try and get rid of that phobia forever. The first thing you would do is to be more mindful and to listen to your own thoughts and reflect on them. If you've been practicing, this should rob them of their power as you become detached and aloof from those thoughts.

But at the same time, you're also going to make a note of them so you can try and change them...

Journaling

Another technique used for the same end is 'journaling'. This involves writing down the feelings as they come to you, or writing them in a journal at the end of the day. That evening routine is coming in handy at this point! See... it all comes together...

Cognitive Restructuring

The next steps all fall under the category of 'cognitive restructuring'. You can think of this as 'reprogramming' yourself...

Thought Challenging

Thought challenging is simple: it means that you're looking at those thoughts you made a note of and now you're challenging them and testing whether or not you really think they're true.

So if you're afraid of public speaking, it may be that you think things like 'I'm going to stutter and everyone will laugh at me!'.

In thought challenging, we're going to deconstruct that belief and see if it really is likely/if it is anything to really be afraid of.

Ask yourself:

- Why would you stutter? Do you normally stutter when you talk?

- Why would people laugh at you? Are people usually that unkind?

- Would *you* laugh if someone had a hard time giving a speech? Or would you be more sympathetic and understanding than that?

Does it matter? You aren't going to see these people again... why does it matter what they think of you?

Ask yourself these things and focus on the fact that the worst case scenario really isn't all that bad. Once you can start doing that, you'll see that there's nothing to be afraid of. You can even repeat a maxim to yourself as a 'positive affirmation':

"It really doesn't matter what these people think of me. It really doesn't matter what these people think of me."

Hypothesis Testing

This is one of the most unpleasant and upsetting treatments that are a part of CBT but it's also by far one of the most immediately effective. The idea is that you're looking at those fears you have and then you're just going to test if they're true.

So in other words, if you're afraid of stuttering when you do public speaking, you're now going to go up on that stage… and you're going to not say anything. You might purposefully stutter. You might say the most awkward thing that comes to mind. You're *testing* the theory that people will laugh.

And guess what? Nine times out of 10 you'll find your imagination was worse than the reality. Now people will just wait politely because that's what people do. Either that or they will laugh… but it won't really matter.

Exposure Therapy

Finally, exposure therapy is just like 're-association'. This just means you're going to face your fear repeatedly until *that* gets desensitized. In the case of public speaking, this might mean that you start attending classes to become a stand-up comic. Scary? Definitely. Effective? You bet.

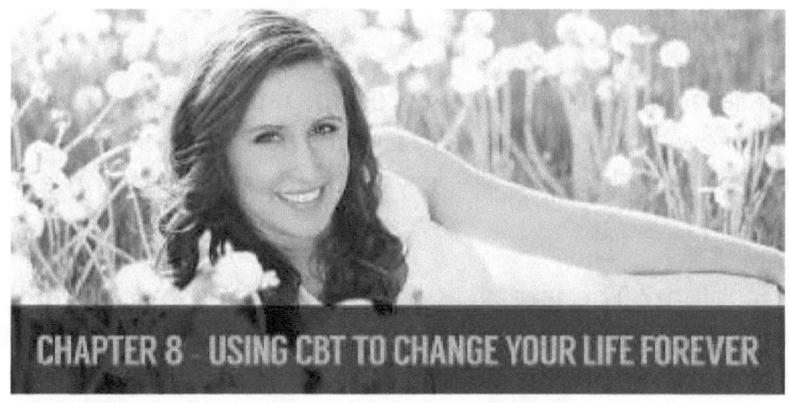

CHAPTER 8 - USING CBT TO CHANGE YOUR LIFE FOREVER

Chapter 8: Using CBT to Change Your Life Forever

The above techniques might sound quite simple, but this is some of the most powerful stuff you will perhaps ever learn. This is all about being more aware of your own mind and once again, taking control of that in order to change the way you want to think and feel.

You can use CBT to overcome any phobia or any problem. If you're afraid of heights, assess *why* and then start to address those fears and to reprogram the way you think about them.

Likewise, if you find that you're not great at meeting women/men, you can likely practice in your mind and force yourself to face those fears.

But you can take CBT further too and impact on other areas of your life. Here are some good examples...

Sleep Soundly

If you're someone who struggles to get to sleep, then you'll know that this can end up impacting every other aspect of your life and leave you tired, stressed and even unhealthy.

The problem? The later it gets, the more stressed and anxious you become. The solution is to apply a little CBT. This time, the focus is going to be on identifying your thought processes and then seeing what would be more useful in that given moment.

The problem is trying to 'force' yourself to sleep. When you do this, you create stress and when you're stressed, you can't sleep.

Instead, try reminding yourself that it doesn't matter if you get to sleep – as long as you're resting. Resting is good for you no matter what, so just lie down and *enjoy* being comfy. Focus on it. You'll be asleep in minutes.

Overcome Anxiety

CBT is incredibly effective for treating anxiety attacks. Somewhat ironically, one of the biggest dangers with panic attacks is that they make us stressed. Because we're stressed *about* anxiety, this makes us become even more stressed and we work ourselves into a fluster that can end with fainting and hyperventilation.

The solution? You have to just acknowledge it for what it is and *allow* it to pass. Say 'this is a panic attack, I must let it run its course' and then just allow it to happen. Go about your business as you normally would and don't try and do anything about it.

You can also do something similar when trying to be less stressed generally – and especially when trying to calm yourself before an interview. Instead of worrying that you're stressed, just remind yourself that stress can be *useful*. Now let yourself.

Gratitude

Something else powerful you can use is to apply a 'gratitude attitude'. This is like CBT, except in this case you're not trying to combat a fear or stress. Instead, you're simply going to change your focus again – and this time you're focusing on what makes you happy and what you're grateful for.

This is a great change because a lot of us are so caught up in everything that's wrong, that we never think about how much is right.

Take a moment at the end of each day and write down the things you are grateful for. Your partner maybe? Your job? Your house? Your dog? The computer game you're playing? There's so *much* to be happy about but a lot of the time we miss it. Take your new ability to change the way you think and focus on it. Suddenly *everything* becomes happier.

Entering Flow

Finally, how about using CBT to enter flow at will?

Remember what we said? Flow is a natural response to what your body and mind deem a highly important stimulus. What defines the importance of a stimulus? Your interpretation of it. So remind yourself why this is important, tell yourself you need to concentrate.

MAKE yourself excited. And engage!

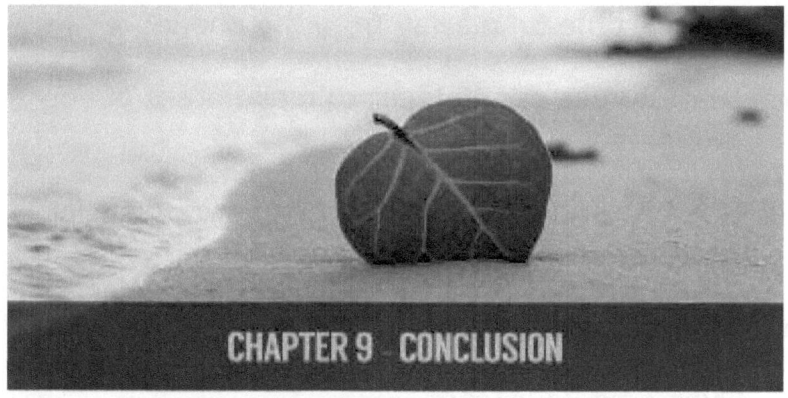

CHAPTER 9 - CONCLUSION

Chapter 9: Conclusion

And there you have it – with that you now know the most powerful and important tools available to you to take back control of your mind.

To recap:

- Practice meditation to learn to calm your mind and shut out concerns

- Learn to meditate on the move and to escape your stresses at will

- Try guided meditation if you struggle

- Make your environment and routine more interesting

- Take up sports and start entering flow

- Stop letting things distract you – have a morning routine

- Spend some time away from the phone

- Learn to use mindfulness to make notes of your thoughts

- Use CBT and cognitive restructuring to develop healthier responses to situations

- Practice gratitude

- Overcome your fears

- Enter flow and focus at will

Now you don't need to change your environment, because you can change the way *you* want to *feel* about it.

Do you want to be stressed and angry? Or happy and inspired? It's a choice!

And once you can do that, you can stop reacting to life and start controlling it. Now you can make life the way *you* want it to be.

It all just takes a little focus...

Cheat Sheet: More Powerful Techniques

In *Calm Mind – Healthy Body*, we discussed in detail the power of taking control of your mind and learning to change the way you think about different situations and events. What we learned was that our experience is really something that happens *within* more than without – and that our happiness, focus and more is all dependent on the way we interpret and react to events rather than those events themselves.

You should now understand this and have the power to use meditation and CBT to overcome those stresses.

But it doesn't end there! In fact, there are countless ways you can change your mind for the better. This cheat sheet will serve as your 'quick guide' to help you learn more!

'Fear Setting'

Fear setting is a concept that comes from author Tim Ferriss and that essentially borrows some key principles from CBT – so you should be familiar with the basics.

Essentially, fear setting is like goal setting – except you're writing down your fears instead of your goals. These are the fears specifically that are *holding you back* from particular goals. So if your goal is to launch your own business, your fears might be:

- What if I'm not successful and I get into debt?

- What if I can't support my family?

- What if my family think I'm reckless and leave me?

- What if I can't get back my old job?

- What if it blows up in my face and everyone laughs at me?

- What if I hate it?

That's step one.

Step two is to write down how likely each of those fears are to become reality and to write down the contingency plans in each scenario – what would you do if that *did* happen?

Essentially, this is just the same as using cognitive restructuring via 'thought challenging' but it's in a more structure manner.

So now you might write:

- What if I'm not successful and I get into debt? – Possible – I can live off savings/look for my old job

- What if I can't support my family? – Unlikely – We can make do off of one salary/I can ask my parents for help/I can get another job

- What if my family think I'm reckless and leave me? – Very unlikely – If it did happen, I should question the loyalty of my family

- What if I can't get back my old job? – Fairly Unlikely – But there are many other jobs I could do. Even if it means working in a supermarket for a while.

- What if it blows up in my face and everyone laughs at me? – Unlikely – I will just say 'at least I tried'

- What if I hate it? – Unlikely – I just change my job back

Suddenly, you've exposed your fears as being not worthy of your consideration. Now you know what you'll do if you do find yourself in those scenarios and you generally have robbed your concerns of the power they might have previously had over you.

And Tim Ferriss takes this technique one step further too by recommending that you write down the *opposite* fear.

What's the opposite fear in this case?

It's:

Staying in the same job forever and never accomplishing my dreams – Likely

Which is *actually* more terrifying?

As you can see, CBT doesn't just apply to every day concerns and phobias – it can even be used to change your motivations and your goals and to help you chase after your dreams!

Visualization

The next trick we're going to look at that you can use to shape your mind the way you want it is 'visualization'. And what we're going to see here is that visualization is actually a far more powerful and integral tool than you may have previously given it credit for.

Embodied Cognition

Embodied cognition teaches us that the way we think about *everything* is linked to the sensations in our bodies and to our senses. That is to say, that the only way we understand words, is by relating it to our physical experience.

When you are born, you don't have any ability to understand English. That is to say that it's not innate and it must be learned. So what is your 'original' language that you think in? What is your brain translating English *into* so that it's native and you can understand it?

The answer is that your brain is converting the language to what it *does* innately understand: experience.

And when it does this, you can actually see the relevant areas of the brain lighting up under a brain scanner as though it were 'happening' to the person. When someone tells you about walking, you imagine walking and the relevant areas of your brain light up to show that you're walking. When someone tells you about a bad day at work, mirror neurons fire as though you're watching someone being shouted at or as though *you're* being shouted at.

In short, we understand by 'simulating' the experience in our brain.

Using Visualization

And this makes visualization incredibly powerful. This is you *actively* simulating situations and as far as your brain is concerned, it's just like it's happening.

This now means you can use visualization in a number of ways.

One of the most common and popular uses for visualization for instance is to go to a 'happy place'. This is one way to find an oasis of calm in a stressful day. All you're simply doing is imagining that you're somewhere that makes you feel relaxed and happy. That might mean that you're sitting in an imaginary field surrounded by the sounds of animals and by beautiful flowers, or it might be that you think back to being in that situation.

At the same time though, this also means that you can use visualization as a tool in CBT. Instead of focussing on the 'words', go deeper and focus on the visualization. Maybe you don't have ruminations that make you nervous to speak in public – maybe it's more like visions!

So correct those visions. Choose how you want it to go and how it will *realistically* go. Visualize it that way and your body will produce the neurotransmitters as though it's really happening – priming you for optimum performance.

Resources

Ready to start making meditation a part of your daily routine? These tools, resources and products can help you to do just that!

Resources

A Guide to Meditation for the Rest of Us
http://www.lifehacker.co.uk/2010/07/20/guide-meditation-rest-us

This is a very good guide to meditation from Lifehacker. Meditation can sometimes seem a bit daunting for those of us who aren't already familiar with it but this article puts it all in layman's terms so anyone can understand it.

CBT Self Help Guide
http://www.getselfhelp.co.uk/cbtstep1.htm

This is a great site that provides a lot of information on CBT and which shows you how to apply it in your own life in order to combat anxiety and stress etc.

Four Hour Workweek Blog
http://fourhourworkweek.com/blog/

We mentioned Tim Ferriss in the book a couple of times. He introduced us to 'fear setting' and also interviewed many famous individuals who explain how they use meditation. You can see all that and more at his blog.

Flow States
http://www.thebioneer.com/neuroscience-of-flow-states/

This is an in-depth post on flow states, what they are and how you can use them in your own life.

Tools

The 4-Hour Workweek Tools
http://fourhourworkweek.com/4-hour-workweek-tools/

This is a list of tools from Tim Ferriss, many of which are very useful for getting on top of your daily concerns and improving your

Headspace

The headspace app is a great app that you can use to trial some guided meditations. Essentially, this is a series of videos that will show you how to get started with meditation in just a few short 'chunks'. The downside is that you have to pay once you get into it but if you want you can just use the free sessions as a jumping off point.

Guided Meditation for Detachment From Over-Thinking
https://www.youtube.com/watch?v=1vx8iUvfyCY

There is no shortage of video on YouTube that can help you to practice meditation. This is just one of many but with that said, it's a very good one and a good place to start. This is a 40+ minute meditation that can help you to understand the benefits of meditation and to leave behind some of those unnecessary worries.

Products

Heartrate Monitor

A heartrate monitor can be a very useful tool for improving your general mood and for getting better at meditation. Meditating should help your heartrate to lower and your blood pressure to do the same. A heartrate monitor thus allows you to see if you're effectively managing to do that or not and also lets you see when you're getting stressed in daily life/how you can combat that stress. This is called 'biofeedback' and it's a powerful tool.

MindWave from NeuroSky
http://store.neurosky.com/

This is an 'EEG' headset. The idea of this is to allow you to use your brainwaves to power apps and also to measure your own concentration, focus and calm. An EEG is an 'electroencephalograph' and is one tool that GPs and psychologists can use to measure brainwaves. Now it is available commercially for the first time and is definitely worth looking into.

Mind Map

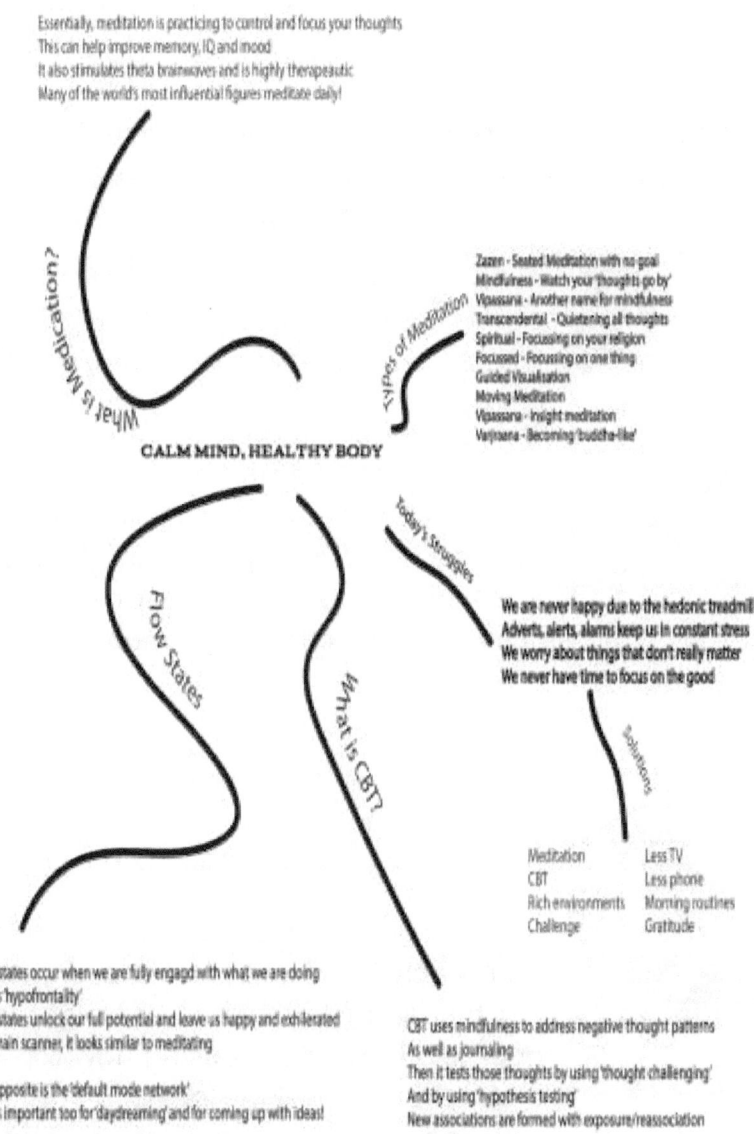

Essentially, meditation is practicing to control and focus your thoughts
This can help improve memory, IQ and mood
It also stimulates theta brainwaves and is highly therapeutic
Many of the world's most influential figures meditate daily!

What is Meditation?

Types of Meditation

Zazen - Seated Meditation with no goal
Mindfulness - Watch your 'thoughts go by'
Vipassana - Another name for mindfulness
Transcendental - Quietening all thoughts
Spiritual - Focussing on your religion
Focussed - Focussing on one thing
Guided Visualisation
Moving Meditation
Vipassana - Insight meditation
Varjrasana - Becoming 'buddha-like'

CALM MIND, HEALTHY BODY

Today's Struggles

We are never happy due to the hedonic treadmill
Adverts, alerts, alarms keep us in constant stress
We worry about things that don't really matter
We never have time to focus on the good

Flow States

What is CBT?

Solutions

Meditation   Less TV
CBT   Less phone
Rich environments   Morning routines
Challenge   Gratitude

Flow states occur when we are fully engagd with what we are doing
This is 'hypofrontality'
Flow states unlock our full potential and leave us happy and exhilerated
In a brain scanner, it looks similar to meditating

The opposite is the 'default mode network'
This is important too for 'daydreaming' and for coming up with ideas!

The key is to be able to choose and activate the best brain state for the situation!

CBT uses mindfulness to address negative thought patterns
As well as journaling
Then it tests those thoughts by using 'thought challenging'
And by using 'hypothesis testing'
New associations are formed with exposure/reassociation

Other Senior Health and Fitness Books by This Author

If you would like to read more about Senior Health and Fitness, here is a list of the titles, CreateSpace links and descriptions:

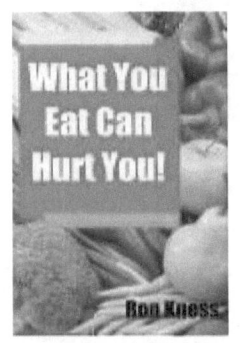

What You Eat Can Hurt You

https://www.createspace.com/4963196

Do you know that certain foods increase your risk for inflammation, disease and illness? It's true! And certain foods can help cure and heal you if you do get sick. Knowing which foods to eat and which ones to avoid empowers you to manage your own health.

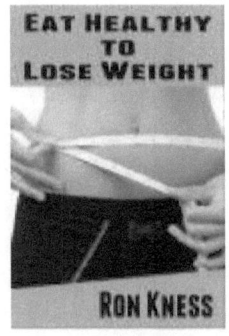

Eat Healthy to Lose Weight

https://www.createspace.com/4962939

As you read through our book, we show you which foods you should and should not be eating to reach your weight loss goal, along with discussing how to maintain your weight loss and stay within a few pounds of your goal weight. Banish the weight you keep gaining back each time by learning how to live a healthy lifestyle.

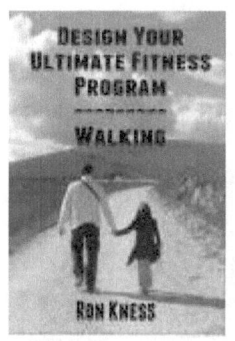

Design Your Ultimate Fitness Program - Walking

https://www.createspace.com/5252272

In my book Design Your Ultimate Fitness Program – Walking, we discuss the considerations that need to be made when designing a custom walking program, along with:
• Equipment needed
• Wearable technology you can use to track your walking
• And how to make walking more challenging

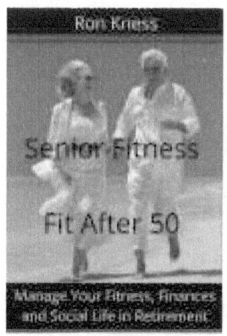

Senior Fitness – Fit After 50: Learn How to Manage Your Fitness, Finances and Social Life in Retirement

https://www.createspace.com/5474751

Inside you will discover answers to your most pressing questions:
• What do I need to know about downsizing my home?
• What are the best tips for staying healthy as you approach your 50's?
• When should I start planning for retirement?
• I am worried about being lonely once I retire, do others feel the same?

• Is it worthwhile to carry two homes during retirement? And more...

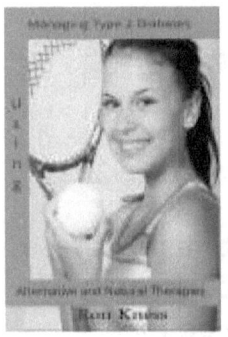

Managing Type 2 Diabetes Using Alternative And Natural Therapies

https://www.createspace.com/5401244

While Type 2 diabetes can be managed medically, there are many alternative natural and holistic methods of therapy and treatment that can further enhance quality of life and minimize the effects of this disease. In this book, I discuss 12 different types, including yoga, reflexology and acupuncture to name just three.

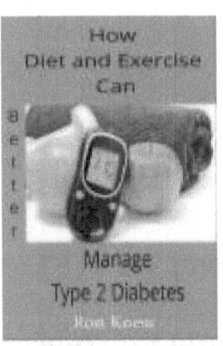

How Diet and Exercise Can Better Manage Type 2 Diabetes

https://www.createspace.com/5404845

Of the different types of diabetes, only Type 2 can be reversed. In my book How Diet and Exercise Can Better Manage Type 2 Diabetes, we reveal the three things you can do to best manage your disease, including:
• Diet
• Exercise
• Weight management

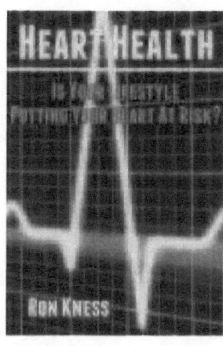

Heart Health: Is Your Lifestyle Putting Your Heart at Risk?

https://www.createspace.com/5464020

In my ebook Is Your Lifestyle Putting Your Heart At Risk? we discuss the six greatest risks to your heart and the lifestyle changes you can make to mitigate them.

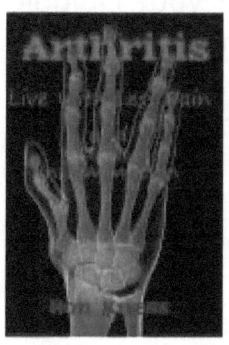

Arthritis – Live Wth Less Pain and Inflammation: Tips and Techniques You Can Use to Lessen the Pain and Inflammation

https://www.createspace.com/5457441

Discover Simple Tips & Information That Will Help Reduce The Painful Symptoms Of Arthritis!

You learn things like:
• Simple and effective information that will help you manage the pain and inflammation that comes along with arthritis, so that you can live an active, full life without debilitating pain.
• The different types of arthritis, their symptoms and how to alleviate their painful side effects.
• The pros and cons of over-the-counter arthritis medications, plus simple tips that will help you know how to choose the right supplements.

• Free, yet effective ways to get relief from arthritis pain and inflammation, so you don't have to suffer anymore. the effects arthritis can have significant impact on your physical and mental well-being, but this books shows you how to overcome its painful symptoms and live life relatively pain free.

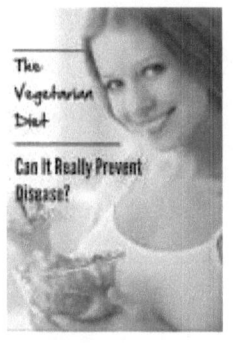

The Vegetarian Diet – Can It Really Prevent Disease?

https://www.createspace.com/5519874

Is a vegetarian diet right for you? Multiple studies have shown over and over that a vegetarian diet goes along way in preventing certain chronic diseases, such as:

• Heart Disease
• Cancer
• Diverticulitis
• Type 2 Diabetes
• Hypertension
• Obesity
• Kidney Failure

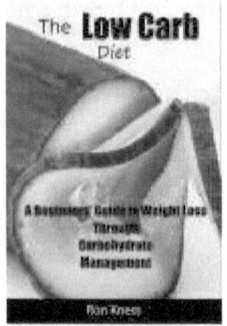

The Low Carb Diet: A Beginner's Guide to Weight Loss Through Carbohydrate Management

https://www.createspace.com/5416348

In my book "The Low-Carb Diet – A Beginners' Guide to Weight Loss Through Carbohydrate Management", I reveal a successful method of losing weight based in part on the amount and type of carbohydrates you consume.

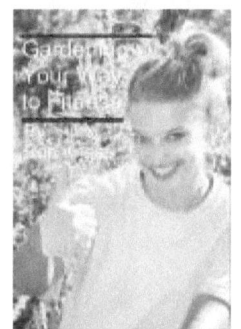

Gardening Your Way to Fitness: The Fun Way to Get Fit and Provide Beauty and Healthful Bounty for Your Family

https://www.createspace.com/5459564

The gym is a great place to stay fit during the colder seasons, but once the temperature turns warmer you want to spend more time outside. Plus, you'll have the benefit of fresh wholesome produce to enjoy by growing vegetables in your backyard garden.

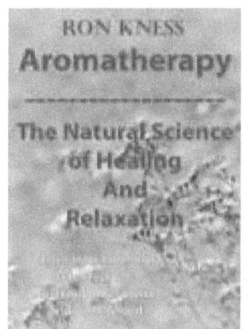

Aromatherapy - The Science of Healing and Relaxation: Learn How Essential Oils Elicit The Relaxation Response And Alter Mood

https://www.createspace.com/5714434

In my book Aromatherapy – The Science of Healing and Relaxation, we reveal the natural holistics methods you can use to heal the body from certain medical issues and to relive stress through relaxation. In particular we talk about:
• Aromatherapy - what it is and how it works

• Essential Oils – how the effects of certain aromas differs from others
• Recipes – how to make your own essential oil combinations

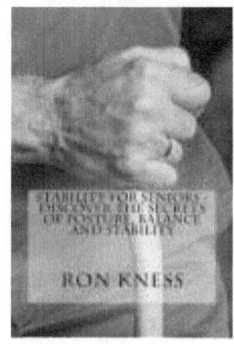

Stability for Seniors: Discover the Secrets of Posture, Balance and Stability

https://www.createspace.com/6096479

Many people sacrifice their health in pursuit of their career. They are so busy making a living that they neglect to make a life. The excuse that they do not have time to exercise is tossed about so frequently that they end up letting their health and fitness slide.

If you are not regularly active, you will have muscular atrophy over time. Your flexibility will decrease. Your core strength will diminish. As time progresses, you will be less limber and more rigid.

This is exactly how people age poorly. It's a process that has snowballed over time.

Only with regular exercise and a healthy diet can you have a body that is fit and has the ability to almost reverse aging.

If you have neglected your health for years and life seems to be a chore now because you can't get around without assistance, do not feel dejected.

You can remedy the situation. You can restore the strength, balance and stamina that you have lost. It is never too late to become what you might have been.

This guide will show you exactly what you need to do to restore your balance, strengthen your core and give you the ability to live life to its fullest. Read how ...

About the Author

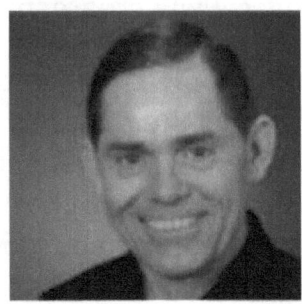

I grew up in Central Minnesota, where my parents owned and operated a fishing resort. Once out of high school I tried a couple of semesters of college, only to quit halfway through the Spring term; I decided at that time that college wasn't for me.

Then I decided to follow my father's previous occupation as an auto mechanic. I graduated from a two-year of vocational training course and worked as a mechanic. While in vocational training, I decided to join the National Guard where I eventually ended up working full-time for 32 years.

So how does all of this relate to writing? In one of my leadership schools, the instructor, who was an English teacher at a juvenile detention center, presented writing to me in a whole new way - a way that started to develop my interest in working with words.

Fast forward about 40 years and I now have over 50 books listed on Amazon for Kindle and CreateSpace.

Besides my own writing, I also ghostwrite ebooks, reports, articles, blogs and do Kindle conversions for my clients on a variety of topics.

Today my wife and I live in Gold Canyon, AZ, where you'll find me happily sitting in my office typing away on my laptop as I work on my next book or ghostwriting project . . . that is if we are not traveling on a cruise ship - our new-found mode of travel.